Teachers of Healing and Wholeness

Hippocrates

Also in this series

Other titles in preparation

Teachers of Healing and Wholeness

Hippocrates
The Natural Regimen

ARTHUR JAMES
BERKHAMSTED

First published in Great Britain by
ARTHUR JAMES LTD
70 Cross Oak Road
Berkhamsted
Hertfordshire HP4 3HZ

A catalogue record for this book is available from
the British Library.

ISBN 0 85305 411 8

Typeset in Monotype Columbus by
Strathmore Publishing Services, London N7

Printed in Great Britain at
Ipswich Book Company, Ipswich, Suffolk

Contents

• • • • • • • • •

Series Introduction
· · · · · · · · · · · · · · · · · · ·

At a time when the limitations of modern medicine are becoming clear, growing numbers of people are looking back to older approaches to healing and wholeness. The series aims to make available to the general reader original writings of the great teachers, from every part of the world and from every period of history.

The particular insights of the different teachers vary, and each has special wisdom for us to hear. Yet various themes recur. They all stress the unity of the spiritual and physical aspects of human nature, and therefore the need to care for the whole person. They emphasise the importance of the way we conduct our daily lives, both to prevent and to cure illness. And they seek to harness the latent powers of self-healing.

None of the healers in this series claimed to be infallible; all saw themselves as explorers. Thus none asked for uncritical trust; they regarded themselves as partners with those who listened to their words. In reading their works today we should see ourselves as partners, reflecting on what they say, and taking such advice as we think is right.

Introduction

• • • • • • • • • • • •

Hippocrates is revered as 'father' of their discipline, both by orthodox medical practitioners and by many who use alternative methods of healing. Hippocrates is credited with taking medicine out of the hands of priests and magicians, and establishing it as a science based on experiment and observation: hence his status amongst western doctors and researchers who seek to follow a strict scientific code. Yet Hippocrates was sceptical of drugs, and saw the correct diet, appropriate exercise, and the right environment as the essential means of healing – so in recent decades those looking for more natural means of promoting and preserving good health have looked to him for inspiration.

Almost nothing is known about the life of Hippocrates. According to Plato and Aristotle, who recognised his greatness, he was born on the island of Cos in about 460 BC, and became famous as an itinerant healer. They also mention that he taught the science of healing to others, charging them a fee. Beyond this they are silent. But after his death – probably in Thessaly in about 370 BC – his name shone ever brighter, eclipsing other healers of the period who were developing similar methods. As a result, facts were embellished and legends created. For example, in Macedonia he is said to have cured the king of a wasting disease by recognising that its cause was psychological rather than physical. Elsewhere in Abdera he supposedly cured a man of madness by discerning its physical origin, and prescribing a change of diet.

Equal uncertainty surrounds the authorship of works traditionally ascribed to him. Some time after his death a number of works were put together under the title 'Hippocratic Corpus'. Judging by both style and content, a number of authors are represented in this Corpus; and scholars have found it impossible to detect the pen of Hippocrates himself. To confuse matters further, in the following centuries other treatises were added. Nonetheless all the works in the Corpus have a common approach to healing, with similar ideas frequently repeated; so one can speak quite properly of a Hippocratic 'school' of healing.

The Hippocratic school distinguishes two kinds of illness. Firstly there are general illnesses which a large number of people contract at the same time; these are caused by some aspect of the environment. Secondly there are particular diseases which individuals contract, due to disturbances or imbalances in the body. Thus the science of healing has two aspects. As far as possible the environment must be made conducive to good health; and insofar as this is impossible, the individual must compensate for its deficiencies. And the individual's daily routine should promote harmony and balance within the body.

The part of daily routine which receives the strongest emphasis is diet; and the various treatises are packed with nutritional advice. Today we are apt to imagine that our lists of vitamins, proteins and minerals encompass all we need to know about nutrition; but the continuing flow of new discoveries suggests that our ignorance may still exceed our knowledge. The Hippocratic approach is based on trying to observe what is natural: just as other creatures thrive if they eat and drink what Nature intends, so will the human species. And this leads to a profound respect for traditional dietary wisdom, since our ancestors over thousands of years have learnt from experience which foods suit the human body and which do not. In terms of food itself, the Hippocratic school reaches conclusions remarkably similar to those of modern nutritional science. But it stresses also the importance of regular meal-times.

The Hippocratic School described and codified a wide range of distinct diseases; and the case histories that were written down remain of great interest to medical historians. The Hippocratic healers possessed a refreshing humility, recognising that with most illnesses medical intervention is at best useless and at worst downright harmful; the illness must simply run its course. They did, however, see the importance of quite simple treatments, like warm poultices, massage, hot baths and extra sleep. And they offered basic advice for common ailments, such as catarrh, diarrhoea, sciatica, arthritis, inflamed wounds, hiccups and, most importantly, chronic pain.

The Hippocratic Corpus includes two rather surprising treatises. The first is an analysis of dreams, as a method of medical prognosis. Various images and events that occur in dreams are listed; and a particular illness is ascribed to each. This might appear as a lapse into the magical approach to medicine which the Hippocratic healers were rejecting. Yet the claim implicit in the treatise is that dreams have proven themselves to be accurate predictors of disease. The second is a description and advice about sexual intercourse. Although some of the anatomical details – such as that sperm is made up from fluids taken from the entire body – are inaccurate, the treatise is remarkable in presenting the man and woman as equal partners, both in the process of conception and in the pleasure enjoyed. It also contains a rather crude method of contraception; but here too its importance is in the underlying attitude, that sex is as much for mutual enjoyment as for procreation.

Although the famous Hippocratic oath is for healers, and although the case histories and some of the treatises are written for the medical experts of the day, the emphasis throughout the Hippocratic Corpus is on self-treatment. Healing can only be achieved and good health preserved if individuals follow the right pattern of diet and exercise, and live in a healthy environment. Thus, as the treatises frequently repeat, the right mental attitude is a vital ingredient for health and healing. And even when a healer is called in, the healer can only succeed with the full and active cooperation of the patient – and of the patient's relatives and friends. So today the Hippocratic Corpus should not merely be studied by doctors and medical historians; all of us can benefit hugely from its time-honoured wisdom.

I

Principles of Healing
••••••••••••••••••••••••

Oath

I will use my power to help the sick to the best of my ability and judgement; I will refrain from harming or doing wrong to any person by it.

I will not give a fatal draught to those who ask, nor will I suggest such a course. I will not help a woman to abort a foetus.

I will be chaste and devout in my life and in my actions.

When I visit a house, my purpose will be to help the sick, and never to cause harm or injury. I will not abuse my position to indulge in sexual contacts with other men or women.

Whenever I see or hear things which should not be divulged, I will keep them secret and tell no one.

If I observe this oath and do not violate it, may I prosper both in my life and in my profession, earning the respect of all people.

Self-treatment

Those who are wise realise that good health is their most precious possession. Thus they should learn how to treat their illnesses by their own judgement.

Factors to Consider

In studying the science of healing we must consider the seasons of the year, and the differences between them. We must observe the warm and the cold winds, both those which are common to every region, and those peculiar to a particular locality. We must not forget the effect of water on people's health: whether it is marshy and soft, whether it is hard because it flows over rocky ground, or whether it is salty. And lastly we must look at people's way of life: whether they are heavy eaters and drinkers, and take little exercise; or whether they enjoy exercise, and eat and drink in moderation.

Two Kinds of Disease

Some diseases are caused by the manner of life that we lead; others by the air we breathe. This distinction can easily be demonstrated. When a large number of people all catch the same disease at the same time, the cause is clearly something common to all; and this must be in the air they breathe. The individual's bodily habits and condition cannot be responsible because the disease attacks young and old, men and women, those who drink wine and those who only drink water, those who eat barley-cakes as well as those who only eat bread, those who take much exercise and those who are sedentary, and so on. But when many different diseases appear at the same time, clearly the cause lies in each individual's pattern of life.

Epidemics

Epidemics of a particular disease, caused by some morbid substance within the air we breathe, should be combatted by reducing the quantity of food and drink consumed, so that the body is carrying as little weight as possible. This reduction should not be made quickly, since a sudden change may cause a further disease; the reduction should be gradual. A lighter body does not require so much air, so less of the morbid substance will be inhaled. It is also advisable, wherever practicable, to move away from the area of the epidemic to where the air is different.

Treatment by Opposites

Diseases caused by over-eating are cured by fasting; those caused by starvation are cured by feeding up. Diseases caused by excessive exertion are cured by rest; those caused by indolence are cured by exertion. Thus we can infer a general principle, that a disease caused by a person's pattern of life should be treated by the opposite of its cause. With such diseases, therefore, the unhealthy aspect of a person's pattern of life must be carefully discerned, taking into account the person's age and appearance, and also the season of the year. Then the correct treatment can be worked out.

Balance and Disturbance

Those who are naturally stout have a constitution which is finely balanced, and so can be easily disturbed; they remain at the peak of their powers only for a short period. Those who are naturally lean have a more robust constitution which is rarely disturbed; they remain at the peak of their powers for a much longer period.

Those constitutions which react rapidly and severely to changes in routine are weak. A weak constitution is prone to sickness, and a sick person is made even weaker by disruption to the normal pattern of life.

It is dangerous to make sudden changes in diet or in any other aspect of life. All sudden changes are inimical to human nature. When people should change their diet or some other aspect of life, in order to improve their health, they should proceed gradually, little by little.

Athletes should not train their bodies to an extreme state of fitness. Their bodies cannot remain in that state; and, since they cannot get better, they can only change for the worse. For this reason athletes should immediately reduce their state of fitness, so their bodies can regain equilibrium. Also athletes should not allow their bodies to become too thin, because this too cannot be sustained; they should attain their natural weight, whatever that may be.

Cold and Heat

When cold and heat are present together in the body, they are harmless, because heat is tempered by cold and cold by heat. When the two are separated from each other, then they become harmful. But happily when the body is chilled, warmth is spontaneously generated by the body itself, so there is no need to take special measures; this is true for both the healthy and the sick. For example, if a healthy man cools himself by taking a cold bath, then the cooler his body becomes, the warmer he feels as he puts on his clothes again. Similarly, if a man warms himself thoroughly with a hot bath or sitting by a fire, and then goes into a cool place, that place feels much colder than before and he starts to shiver. The same is true in more extreme situations. If people get their feet frozen by walking through snow, then later, when they are snug in bed, their feet have a burning sensation. Similarly, when people sweat with fever they feel much colder than if they had no fever. We may conclude that heat and cold can cause no great harm to the body, since invariably the presence of one quickly stimulates the appearance of the other, removing any ill effects.

Drugs

Use drugs only very seldom, and then at the early stage of a disease. Before using drugs, ensure that you fully understand the disease, so that you can be sure which drugs are appropriate.

When a disease has reached its crisis, or when the crisis has just passed, do not disturb the sick person with drugs or stimulants. Let the sick person recover naturally.

State of Mind

In every disease a healthy state of mind and a good appetite is beneficial. But if a person becomes depressed, or loses interest in food, the disease is likely to get worse.

The source of our pleasure, merriment, laughter and amusement, as well as our grief, pain, anxiety and tears, is the brain. It is the organ which enables us to think, see and hear; and to distinguish the ugly and the beautiful, the bad and the good, the pleasant and the unpleasant. The brain is also the seat of madness and delirium, and of the fears and terrors which assail us at night. It contains the cause of insomnia and sleepwalking. All mental and emotional problems result from imbalance and disharmony in the brain.

Of all organs the brain is most sensitive to environmental factors, because it perceives its environment directly through the five senses. Thus an unhealthy environment, or sudden changes in the environment, are likely to cause mental problems. The cure for diseases of the brain must, therefore, be sought in the environment; healing comes through making the right environmental changes.

Cooperation

Life is short, science is long; opportunity is elusive, experiment is dangerous, judgement is difficult. It is not sufficient for the physician to act; but those who are sick, as well as relatives and friends, must play their part as well. Also circumstances must be favourable.

Diet and Exercise
• • • • • • • • • • • • • • • • •

Using and Replenishing

Food and exercise possess opposite qualities, yet together they promote good health. Exercise uses up energy, while food and drink replenish it. People should find which forms of exercise best suit their bodies, improving their strength; and they should adjust the amount of food they eat to the amount of exercise they take.

Development of Diet

Our present diet would not have been developed if the food and drink which suits the ox, the horse and other animals also suited humans. Animals grow and thrive on the fruits, vegetables and grass which the earth produces naturally. Originally humans lived on the same raw food. But their stomachs could not digest it properly, and so they suffered many diseases. Thus our primitive ancestors sought food suitable to their bodies, and so discovered what we now eat. They experimented with various forms of cooking, and with mixing one item with another, in order to find foods from which their stomachs could draw nourishment. This process of experiment and discovery, to find a diet which reduces sickness and promotes health, is what we call the science of healing.

Preparing Food

The power of foods to disturb the body, or to promote harmony, is affected by the way in which they are prepared. Strong foods should be boiled. Foods which are excessively moist should be grilled or roasted. Dry foods should be soaked and boiled, as should very salty foods. Bitter and sharp foods should be mixed with sweet ones. Astringent foods should be mixed with oily ones. Food should always be fresh, rather than stale.

Diet Through the Seasons

During winter people should eat more and drink less. The drink should be wine with only a little water. They should eat bread rather than barley-cake; their meat and fish should be roasted; and their vegetables well cooked. This diet will keep the body warm and dry.

When spring comes people should eat less and drink more. They should dilute their wine with a greater amount of water. They should eat fewer cereals, and substitute barley-cake for bread. Meat should be reduced, and it should be boiled rather than roasted. More vegetables should be eaten, and some may be eaten raw. This change should happen gradually as the atmosphere becomes warmer.

During summer the barley-cake should be soft and moist, all meat should be boiled, many raw vegetables should be eaten, and wine diluted with large amounts of water. This will keep the body cool and moist.

When autumn comes this process should be reversed, until the winter diet is resumed.

Virtue of Simple Food

In our food there exists saltiness, bitterness, sweetness, sharpness, stringency, flabbiness and numerous other qualities, each with its own influence and strength. When these qualities are properly mixed and balanced with each other, we barely notice them, and they do no harm. But when one is separated out and stands alone, we notice it, and it causes damage. The foods which do harm to us all have one dominant quality: they are excessively bitter, or sweet, or sharp, or whatever. Those things which form the basic human diet, such as bread and barley-cakes, have no dominant or strange taste; whereas those dishes which are designed to give intense pleasure emphasise some particular quality. We can conclude that simple foods, in which the different qualities are well mixed, give the greatest nourishment and strength, and are least likely to cause sickness.

Meal Times

Some like to dine once a day, and so make this their habit. Others prefer to eat twice, once at noon and again in the evening. It makes little difference to most people's health whether they have one meal a day or two. But there are some who, if they break their custom, quickly become ill. If a person normally only eats in the evening, and then on a particular occasion eats at midday, the immediate result may be great drowsiness and dryness of the mouth. If that person later has a meal in the evening, terrible indigestion may follow – even if the amount consumed at both meals has been modest. Similarly, if a person normally eats at noon, and then for some reason misses that meal, the immediate result may be faintness and dizziness, with a sinking feeling in the stomach. When that person finally sits down to eat in the evening, food will seem distasteful; and sleep that night will be poor, disturbed by violent nightmares.

If for some reason a person has a meal at an unusual time, the person should rest after the meal. In winter the rest should be in a warm place to avoid shivering; and in summer in a cool place to avoid sweating. If sleep will not come, the person should rise and take a long slow stroll. At the next meal the person should eat very sparingly.

Avoidance of Sudden Change

Since sudden changes in diet can have a marked effect on healthy people, it is hardly surprising that dietary changes can cause great damage to the sick. It is generally better for sick people to have less of what they normally eat, rather than to alter completely their diet. Similarly if people are accustomed to two meals a day, they should continue to eat at their habitual times when they are sick; and the same applies to those who eat only once a day.

Over-eating and Slimming

When people start to eat too much, the symptoms are

pleasant. They sleep longer at night, and may also sleep more during the day, because their bodies are moist and restful. But soon the surfeit of food disturbs the body and the soul. They no longer feel relaxed, and they frequently wake during the night; and their dreams become nasty and frightening. They feel aches in their flesh, as if they had over-exerted themselves; and, deluding themselves that they are indeed exercising too much, they may become even more indolent and self-indulgent. They may also bathe too frequently, in order to ease the aches; and excessive bathing combined with over-eating can cause pneumonia. A further symptom is that after sexual intercourse they feel utterly exhausted, barely able to move.

It is vital to act before pneumonia and other serious diseases attack. People who have been eating too much should reduce their diet. They may eat bread which is still warm, and vegetables such as leeks and onions; they should have little meat. They should also eat only once a day, preferably in the evening. They should take frequent, vigorous exercise; and afterwards they should rub oil into their bodies. When there are pangs of hunger, the person may eat figs, as these are an excellent laxative.

Diet for Healing

If the food and drink which suited the sick were the same as that which suited the health, there would be no need for the science of healing. The reason why this science is necessary is because the sick have different dietary needs from the healthy.

There are some who eat and drink the same things when they are ill as they do when they are healthy. They do not abstain from anything, but consume just what they want. When the science of healing began, the sick were advised simply to reduce the quantity of food they ate. But it soon became clear that, while some were helped by this, others were not; indeed some could not digest even small quantities of normal food. So gruel was invented, in which normal foods are mixed with water and cooked at great length, to aid the digestive process.

Only during the most acute phase of a disease, when pain is most severe, should the sick person eat sparingly. At other times the diet should be more substantial; and after the acute phase the amount eaten should increase gradually as the severity of the disease decreases.

It is better for a sick person to eat and drink things which they enjoy, even if these things are less suitable, than to struggle with food and drink which is more suitable but which they dislike.

Bread

The body reacts differently to bread according to the way in which the bread has been prepared: whether white or brown flour has been used; whether the wheat was winnowed or unwinnowed; whether it was mixed with much water or a little, whether it was baked at a high temperature or a low temperature – and so on. The same is true in the preparation of barley meal. The influence of each process is significant, causing the bread to react differently on the body which consumes it. The knowledge we acquire by observing these different reactions is vital to the preservation of health and the curing of disease.

Bread made with the bran still in the flour is an excellent laxative. Bread should not be fried in oil, as this overheats the body and produces wind.

Gruel

Gruel made from barley is a most suitable food for those who are acutely sick. It is smooth, soft and soothing; it is slippery, and so can be easily swallowed; and it quenches thirst. It contains nothing that will cause constipation or serious rumbling. And it does not swell up in the stomach, because it swells to its maximum bulk as it is cooked.

If the disease causes dryness, a drink of either mead or wine should be taken before the gruel; the patient should not consume extra gruel to quench the thirst.

As an alternative to gruel made from barley, a sick person may consume gruel made from lentils. This is especially helpful for disease of the heart. To the lentils add cummin and oil, and either salt or honey.

The person who is recovering from sickness should only have gruel so long as there is no appetite for solid food. But once the person is able and willing to eat normally, gruel should be abandoned in favour of solid food.

Wine

Children should be given wine which has been greatly diluted, and it should not be cold. The wine should be of a kind which is least likely to cause wind and distension of the stomach. This will help prevent convulsions, and enable them to grown strongly and develop good complexions.

Dark, harsh wines do not pass well; and they dehydrate the body, absorbing its moisture. Soft, dark wines pass better, but cause flatulence; the same is true of sweet, dark wines. Harsh white wines pass better, and are less liable to dehydrate the body. Thin, sweet white wines pass best; they also cool and moisten the body.

Milk and Cheese

Milk should not be drunk by those suffering from headaches. It is bad, too, for those with high fever; for those whose bellies are distended and full of rumbling; for those with chronic thirst; and for those losing blood in the stools. Milk is good for those with a prolonged low fever; and for those who have become very thin.

Cheese is strong, nourishing, heating and binding. It is strong because it is made from milk; it is nourishing because milk is designed to nourish animals which are newly-born; it heats the body because it contains fat; it is binding because it is coagulated with fig juice or rennet.

Excessive consumption of foods that are rich and fat, such as cheese, put an undue strain on the digestive system. They cause colic, flatulence and heaviness.

Vegetables, Herbs and Fruits

Garlic warms the body, but dulls the sight; as does onion. The leek is good for the bladder, and also stops heartburn; but you must eat it last, at the end of a meal. The radish is bad for arthritis, and is hard to digest. Coriander, when eaten at the end of a meal, helps sleep. Lettuce cools the body. Nettles purge and purify the body. Mint warms the body, and stops vomiting; if eaten too often it can prevent erections. Cabbage is a laxative, and also reduces flatulence; beetroot has the same qualities. The turnip both warms and moistens the body.

Marjoram warms the body, and purges it; as does savoury. Thyme is effective in clearing the head of phlegm; hyssop is also useful in this way. Clover and fennel are good diuretics.

Fruit generally relaxes the body; and it is more relaxing when it is fresh than when it is dry. Ripe pears moisten the body and pass easily; hard pears can be binding. Apples are hard to digest; but apple juice helps to stop vomiting. Pomegranate juice is a laxative, but may over-heat the internal organs. Grapes are warm and moisten the body, especially white grapes. Almonds are highly nutritious, as are all kinds of nuts; but too many nuts can cause flatulence.

Forms of Exercise

Walking is the most natural form of exercise; but it can jar and disturb the body. A walk after dinner helps to prevent the stomach growing fat. Walks in the early morning make the faculties of seeing and hearing brighter and clearer, and also relax the bowels.

Running should be increased gradually. It heats and dissolves the flesh, and relaxes the whole body. It is especially beneficial to big eaters. It should be done in winter, not in summer.

Swinging the arms is a dangerous form of exercise as it causes sprains.

Dangers of Exercise

Fatigue from exercise causes pain. Those who are out of training suffer these pains after the slightest exertion. Trained bodies feel fatigue pains after unusual exercises, or after excessive exercise. Fatigue pains can be eased in various ways: taking a hot bath; going on a gentle walk; rubbing oil into the painful area; lying on a soft bed; and drinking a soft, light wine, diluted with water. When suffering fatigue pains a person should also have a meal, eating slowly, with a series of small courses, and with a long interval between each.

Those who find that exercise causes diarrhoea, and pass undigested stools, should cut their exercise by at least a third, and also halve the amount of food they consume. The diet, while the diarrhoea lasts, should be bread boiled for a long period, and then crumbled into wine. They should also only eat once a day, to give their bellies the best chance of digesting the food they have taken. This sort of diarrhoea is most common in those who are especially stout; the exercise compresses their vessels, and so inhibits digestion.

3
Environment
• • • • • • • • • • •

Winds

Let us consider first a district which is sheltered from northerly winds, but is exposed to warm winds from the south. Water will be plentiful, but it will mainly be brackish surface water, warm in the summer and cold in the winter. The inhabitants of such a place will have moist heads full of phlegm; this will flow down from the head and disturb their inner organs. Their constitutions will usually be flabby, and they will need to eat wisely and follow a strict routine if they are to avoid sickness.

Consider now a district in the opposite situation, sheltered from the south but with cold prevailing winds from the north. The water will be hard and cold. The people will therefore tend to be lean and sturdy, prone to constipation but with strong chests. They will have more trouble with bile than with phlegm; so they will have sound, hard heads, but suffer frequently from abscesses. They will have good appetites, but little desire for wine.

Those districts facing east are likely to be the healthiest. They do not face such extremes of heat and cold as those facing north and south. The water is generally clear, sweet-smelling and soft; this is because the early morning sunshine distils dew from the morning mist. The people mostly have good complexions, loud and clear voices, and robust temperaments. The diseases in such districts are few, and usually not severe.

The districts facing west, sheltered from the easterly winds and also from the warm south winds, are the least healthy. The water is not clear; this is because the air holds the early morning mist, so takes away the water's sparkle. In summer hot, moist breezes blow ,which burn the people. This gives them poor complexions, their voices are thick and hoarse, and they are prone to all manner of diseases. Not even the northerly gales reach such districts to blow away the damp air.

South winds cause deafness, blurred vision, headaches, sluggishness and lack of energy. North winds bring coughs, sore throats, constipation, difficulties in passing urine, and pains in the side and breast.

Seasons

If the winter is wet and mild with southerly winds, and

this is followed by a cold, dry spring with the wind in the north, people become full of phlegm. They are prone to catarrh in the head, which may spread to the lungs. And if the phlegm flows down into the stomach, people can suffer from dysentery. Amongst old people this excessive phlegm can prove fatal.

If the summer is dry, diseases are soon healed; but if it is wet, diseases last a long time, and breaks in the skin easily turn sore. If a dry summer with a northerly wind is followed by a wet autumn with a southerly wind, then through the winter people will be prone to headaches, hoarseness and a running nose.

It is necessary to take precautions against great changes in the weather. The most dangerous times are the two solstices, especially mid-summer, and the two equinoxes, especially autumn.

The changes of the seasons are especially likely to induce diseases, as are great changes from heat to cold, or cold to heat, in any season.

When the weather is seasonable, and the crops ripen at the expected times, diseases are regular in their appearance, and easily reach their crises. When the weather is unseasonable, diseases are unusual in their appearance, and their crises are difficult.

In the autumn diseases tend to be most acute and dangerous. The spring is the healthiest time of the year.

Water

Water plays a vital role in human health. Stagnant water from marshes and lakes is warm and thick in the summer; in winter it is cold, and is also made muddy from rain running off the surrounding land. Thus stagnant water tends to produce phlegm and hoarseness. People who drink such water usually age and die prematurely.

Water from rock springs is hard, containing various metals such as iron, copper, silver, gold or alum. This water is difficult to pass, and also tends to cause constipation.

The best water comes from high ground, and hills covered in earth. This water is sweet and clean. It is cool in summer and warm in winter because it comes from deep springs. Especially good is water which flows towards the east, or, better still, towards the north-east, because it is very sparkling, sweet-smelling and light.

A person who is in good and robust health need not distinguish between one kind of water and another, but can drink whatever is at hand. But the sick person must be more careful. If the stomach is hard and liable to become inflamed, the sweetest, lightest and most sparkling waters are best. If the stomach is soft, moist and full of phlegm, the hard, salty waters are best, since these will dry up the stomach. For cooking, soft water should be used, as food cooked in soft water relaxes the stomach.

Temperature

Cold is bad for the bones, teeth, nerves, brain and spinal cord; heat is good for these parts of the body.

Cold water should be applied to lacerations of the skin, as it helps to stop the bleeding. Do not apply it to the actual spot where the bleeding occurs, but to the skin nearby.

Cold substances such as snow and ice are harmful to the chest. They cause coughs and discharges of phlegm.

Warmth is helpful in the treatment of ulcers, as it softens and dries the skin, and relieves pain. Warm substances applied to the head relieve headaches. Warmth is also valuable in the treatment of broken bones.

4
Illness and Treatments
· ·

Baths

Bathing is beneficial to most who are sick. Even if not taken in the right way a bath can do little harm. Plenty of water should be used, and there should be no draughts. Baths should be frequent, but not excessively so. It is better not to be rubbed down with soap; but some soap can be added to the water. The sick person should not have to go too far for a bath, and the tub should have low sides so it is easy to climb in and out. The sick person should lie quietly in the bath, with other people pouring the water on the body. A sponge rather than a scraper should be used to clean the skin. Afterwards the body should be anointed with oil while the skin is still slightly wet. On no account should the sick person become chilled. Do not bathe shortly after food or drink; and do not eat or drink shortly after a bath. The decision whether to bathe or not should rest mainly with the sick person; the sick person is in the best position to judge its benefits.

Sleep

Sleep after a meal both aids digestion, and also enables the nourishment to spread across the body. Lack of sleep prevents the body receiving the nourishment from the food it has consumed.

Where sleep makes a disease worse, the disease is very serious. Where sleep is beneficial, the disease is less dangerous. Both sleep and wakefulness are bad if they exceed their due proportion.

When people are sick they should try to follow their normal pattern of sleep, spending the day awake and the night asleep. If more sleep is needed, it is best that the sleep is taken in the late morning or early afternoon. If pain or distress keeps a person awake, this may cause delirium.

Pain

As soon as there is pain, a person should rest; this will help to restore the bodily disturbances which cause the pain.

Those who are accustomed to bearing pain, even if they are old and weak, are less worn down by it than the young and strong which are unaccustomed.

A pain in any part of the body is eased by the application of heat. Hot water should be put in a skin or bladder, or in an urn made of bronze or earthware. A damp cloth or sponge should be put against the skin for comfort; and then the vessel of hot water placed on top. The hot vessel should itself be covered so that it remains hot longer.

If there is a pain in the head, the head should be warmed by being washed in hot water. This may induce the person to sneeze, which may further ease the pain. While the pain continues, the person should not have a heavy meal, but should eat sparingly. And on no account should wine be drunk until the pain has fully disappeared.

To ease pain in the back, boil celery and fennel bark in water, and then drink the water. Afterwards drink diluted white wine. Also wash the place where the pain is located in hot water; and then keep a warm poultice on the place.

Massage

Massage warms the flesh and stimulates it. It compresses the flesh, and in this way draws nourishment to it. Massage also drives stale breath out of the body.

Feeding Up

If people become thin over a long period of time, they should feed themselves up slowly. But when the wasting has come in a short time, they should feed themselves up quickly.

Catarrh

If after a common cold the nose remains congested, and the complexion remains pallid, action should be taken; letting matters drift can cause considerable damage. When the person is at rest the mucus becomes thicker and the nasal passages more congested – which is why the problem is greatest after dinner or after sleep. But when the person is warmed by exercise, the mucus thins, and the nose becomes less congested. Thus the person must take more vigorous exercise, not to the point of becoming fatigued, but in order to warm thoroughly the whole body. Each act of vigorous exercise should be followed by a warm bath. The person should also flush out the mouth and throat at least once a day with a harsh, astringent wine – being careful not to swallow any.

Diarrhoea

Diarrhoea can cause great weakness: although the person may eat a normal amount, the food is not digested. The treatment is to fast, eating nothing, so that the digestive system can relax completely. No wine should be taken; but the juice of white grapes may be drunk to quench the thirst. The person may also drink the juice obtained when lentils or beans are cooked.

Wounds

When the skin has been cut, and especially if the wound has been inflamed, a plaster made from beet should be put on it. The plaster may also be made from celery, olive leaves, fig leaves or sweet pomegranate. The plaster should first be boiled. The plaster should not be applied until it has completely cooled. Under no circumstances should fat be applied to a wound, as this will worsen the inflammation. However, once the wound has begun to heal, fat or oil may be rubbed gently into the new tissue, to aid its growth.

Sciatica and Arthritis

Sciatica is greatly eased by warm baths, and by applying heat to the area of pain.

Arthritis is eased by cold baths, and by applying coolness to the joints which cause pain. Drinking boiled milk can also help.

Hiccups

To cure hiccups, drink vinegar and honey. Boil the vinegar and honey separately, and then mix them. This may be supplemented by a gruel made with barley, to which a little honey has been added. And if hiccups persist, strong white wine should be taken.

5
Dreams
· · · · · · · ·

The Soul's Perception

To understand the meaning of dreams, and the signs which occur within them, is very valuable for many purposes. When the body is awake, the soul is not controlling itself; it is split into a number of parts, each devoted to some particular bodily function such as hearing, vision, touch, limb movement and so on. But when the body is at rest, the soul rises up and becomes its own mentor. The sleeping body receives no sensation, but the soul perceives everything: it has its own eyes and ears, it can walk, it can feel pain, and it can think. In short, during sleep the soul becomes both a body and a soul in itself.

Varieties of Dreams

There are various kinds of dreams. There are dreams which are simply a continuation of the person's day-time actions and thoughts; events in the dream occur as if the body were awake. These dreams indicate that the person is in a healthy condition, without cause for anxiety or depression. But when the thoughts and actions of dreams are quite different from daytime events, and especially when these conflicts between the dreams and other people, these show that the body and soul are disturbed. The seriousness of the conflict in the dreams indicate the seriousness of the disturbances. The person should have only a light diet for at least five days, should have a brisk walk early in the morning, and should do vigorous exercises in the gym; it is also good to exercise the voice. All this will help calm the disturbance.

If, however, the violent dreams continue, the person should have long runs, wearing heavy clothes, so the body sweats profusely. The person should also have no breakfast, and to reduce the other meals even further. Moreover normal foods should be replaced by foods which are dry, pungent and bitter.

Signs of Health

There are various images in dreams that indicate a person is in good health, or a sick person is returning to health. These include the dreamer seeing clearly and hearing distinctly; the dreamer walking firmly without stumbling, and running swiftly; the earth appearing smooth and well-tilled, and the trees with bright green leaves and laden with fruit; rivers seeming to flow easily, wild abundant clear water, but without floods; and springs sparkling in the sunlight.

It is also a sign of good health if the dreamer is aware of being well-dressed, with garments that are neither too large nor too small. White garments are especially favourable, as are shoes which are soft and comfortable.

Signs of Sickness

The appearance of monsters in dreams which frighten the dreamer indicate a surfeit of unaccustomed food, or possibly the onset of cholera. The person should have a light diet for five days, consisting of moist, cool food. Some physical exercise is also desirable, as are warm baths; but the person should avoid direct sunlight or excessive cold.

To seem during a dream to be eating one's normal food indicates under-nourishment. The stronger the apparent taste of the food in the dream, the greater is the degree of the deficiency. To seem during a dream to be eating a vast banquet, and yet deriving little enjoyment, indicates a surfeit of nourishment. The same can be inferred when the dreamer is eating loaves made with cheese and honey.

If the dreamer flees in flight from anything, this indicates problems with blood flows in the body, or dehydration. In either case it is wise to cool the body, and also to increase the intake of liquids.

If the dreamer is attacked by enemy soldiers, this may indicate the onset of madness. The best antidotes are plenty of vigourous exercise, a diet of soft food, frequent warm baths, and ample rest. The person should also avoid becoming excessively cold or hot.

If in a dream the dreamer cannot see or hear properly, this indicates some illness in the head. Longer walks in the early morning and after dinner will usually cure the problem. If the dreamer sees trees that are not bearing fruit, this indicates sexual energy is weak. If the trees are losing their leaves, the cause is excessive coldness and moisture in the body; if the tree is flourishing but barren, the cause is excessive heat and dryness. In the former case, the person should have extra heating in the home, and drink less; in the latter, the person should avoid direct sunlight, and drink more.

If in a dream a river is not flowing normally, this indicates problems with the blood. If the amount of water is greater than normal, there is superfluity of blood; if it is less, there is deficiency. If the water is cloudy, there is disturbance in the smooth flow of blood. In each case the cause is insufficient air coming into the body; so the person must learn to breathe more deeply.

If a spring is not flowing properly, this indicates problems with the bladder passing water. In this case a diuretic should be used.

A rough sea in a dream indicates problems in the bowels, causing constipation. A light and gentle laxative should be used.

An earth tremor or the shaking of a house in a dream predicts the onset of sickness in a healthy person; and it predicts the restoration of health in a sick person. With the healthy person it is wise to change the pattern of diet and exercise, as clearly the present pattern is causing disturbance. With the sick person it is wise to continue the present pattern, since the body is changing for the better.

To see land flooded with water, from a river or the sea, is a sign of excess fluid in the body. To dream of diving into a lake, the sea or a river also indicates excess moisture in the body; a period of fasting, vigorous exercise and a dry diet will be beneficial.

To see land that is black and scorched shows that the body is dehydrated. Stop exercise, and do not eat dry, pungent diuretic food. Instead have boiled barley-water and small quantities of light food, together with plenty of diluted white wine; and take frequent baths.

6

Sex

••••

Sperm

The sperm of the man comes from all the fluids in his body; it consists in the most potent part of these fluids, which is secreted from the rest.

Intercourse for the Man

There are veins and nerves which connect every part of the body to the penis. When during intercourse there is gentle friction on the penis, these veins and nerves grow hot and become congested with fluids; as a result a sensation of pleasure and warmth spreads across the body. As the friction on the penis intensifies, and as the man moves his body with increasing vigour, the fluids produce a foam; and this foam is the most potent part of the fluids. The foam then passes through the veins down to the testicles, and then to the penis.

Intercourse for the Woman

When during intercourse the woman's vagina is rubbed, a sensation of warmth and pleasure spreads across her body. Like the man she emits a fluid; this is released into the womb, making it moist, and may flow out if the womb is open wider than normal. She experiences pleasure throughout intercourse, until the man ejaculates. If her sexual desire is strong, she may emit before the man, after which she does not enjoy the same level of pleasure; but more usually her pleasure finishes when the man has ejaculated. Just as cold water poured into boiling water stops the water boiling, so the man's sperm arriving in the womb extinguishes the heat and the pleasure of the woman. Thus the man and the woman reach their peak of heat and pleasure simultaneously.

Sexual Pleasure

The pleasure experienced by a woman during intercourse is less intense than the man's, but lasts longer. The woman experiences a steady level of pleasure throughout intercourse. The man experiences less pleasure at the beginning, but his pleasure at the moment of ejaculation is very high.

Frequent Intercourse

Sexual intercourse warms the body. So it should be more frequent in winter than in summer. It is especially beneficial to older people, whose bodies can become cold.

It is healthy for a woman to have intercourse. Her womb is moistened by intercourse; if the womb becomes dry, it begins to contract, and this may cause pain to the whole body. Also intercourse heats the blood, which makes it flow more easily; this in turn helps to prevent disease.

Conception

The fluids which men and women emit are sometimes strong and sometimes weak. In fact both men and women emit male and female sperm; and the proportion of male and female sperm determines the fluid's strength – the greater is the proportion of male sperm, the stronger is the fluid. If both partners emit strong fluid, the woman will conceive a boy; if both emit weak fluid, she will conceive a girl; if one partner emits strong fluid, and the other weak, it is impossible to predict whether a girl or boy will be conceived.

Contraception

When a woman has intercourse, but does not wish to conceive, she should try to expel the fluids produced by the man and herself as quickly as possible. If, however, she wishes to conceive, she should retain the fluids in her womb. If the woman takes note of when the fluids have been retained, she will know the precise date on which she has conceived.

Nocturnal Emissions

Nocturnal emissions occur when the fluids in the body become unusually warm, and start to produce foam. As this foam passes down to the penis, the man sees visions as though he were having intercourse, and the foam that is emitted is exactly the same as that which is emitted in intercourse.

Bibliography

• • • • • • • • • • • •

HIPPOCRATES *Writings*, trans. Paul Potter. Loeb Classical Library, Harvard University Press, Cambridge, Massachusetts, 1988.

Hippocratic Writings, trans. J. Chadwick and W. N. Mann. Penguin Books, London, 1978.

Teachers of Healing and Wholeness

Also in the series

Andrew Boorde: Healing Through Mirth

Andrew Boorde was a medieval monk who taught that 'mirth' is the chief means to good health. He believed that if they learn to enjoy life to the full, taking appropriate pleasure in every aspect of God's creation, people will remain healthy in both body and mind. In his famous book, *The Dietary of Health* — one of the first medical books written in English — he showed how different foods, drinks and herbs are appropriate for different temperaments and mental conditions. He combined the classical insights of Hippocrates and Galen with the medical folklore of the English countryside to prescribe a pattern of living and eating which peer and peasant alike could follow.

Teachers of Healing and Wholeness

Also in the series

Huang Di: The Balance of Yin and Yang

Huang Di's *Book of Internal Medicine* is probably the oldest book on healing which we still possess – in its original form it may have been composed over four thousand years ago. He was the first to apply the principles of Yin and Yang to human health. And he was the first exponent of acupuncture, the most famous of Chinese healing techniques. He also applied his medical philosophy to sexual matters, giving advice which sexual counsellors today are discovering anew. Thus without doubt his work is of huge historical importance; it challenges modern western readers to look at themselves, physically and mental, with fresh eyes.

Teachers of Healing and Wholeness

Also in the series

Patanjali: The Threads of Yoga

The best-known contribution of Hinduism to the world is Yoga. Today hundreds of thousands of people practise Yoga, attaining a greater degree of mental tranquillity and physical health. And the chief teacher of Yoga was Patanjali, who lived about two thousand years ago. He wrote a series of aphorisms which describe the state of inner harmony, and show how through meditation this state can be achieved. The aphorisms are also intended as foci for meditation, and thus are themselves aids in the practice of Yoga. The form of Yoga taught by Patanjali requires no special physical or spiritual abilities; it is for all and everyone.